Survival Medicine Handbook:
First-aid In Case Of Emergency And Essential Things To Have In Your Medicine Kit

Disclamer: All photos used in this book, including the cover photo were made available under a Attribution-NonCommercial-ShareAlike 2.0 Generic and sourced from Flickr

Table of content

Survival Medicine Handbook: 1
    First-aid In Case Of Emergency And Essential Things To Have In Your Medicine Kit 1
Introduction 3

Chapter 1 – Pack's 4

Chapter 2 – Tools 6

Chapter 3 – Medicine 9

Chapter 4 – Ropes 14

Chapter 5 – Coverage 16

Chapter 6 – Fire 18

Chapter 7 – Food & Water 20

Conclusion 24

FREE Bonus Reminder 25

Survival Medicine Handbook: 1
    First-aid In Case Of Emergency And Essential Things To Have In Your Medicine Kit 1
Introduction 3
Chapter 1 – Pack's 4
Chapter 2 – Tools 6
Chapter 3 – Medicine 9
Chapter 4 – Ropes 14
Chapter 5 – Coverage 16
Chapter 6 – Fire 18
Chapter 7 – Food & Water 20
Conclusion 24
FREE Bonus Reminder 25

Introduction

While the need for medical attention or survival gear can arise in nearly any circumstance, most situations can be treated with the same basic tools and preparations prior to the arrival of medical personnel. With some simple planning, you can stock your kit or pack for just about any circumstance.

A basic emergency kit should not only stock ointments at band aids, but it should include a few tools and items that you may need if you find yourself stranded or away from help. This includes everything from coverage to prevent being ravaged by the elements, to food and tools that can be used to attract attention. In the following pages, you'll find the basic components of assembling that pack as well as tips to insure that you give yourself the maximum chance of survival in just about any situation.

Before you get overwhelmed, though, it's important to start today if you have nothing. Sort through what you have and start from there. A simple water proof Ziploc back with some gauze, alcohol, and band aids is a start. You can build from there once you've laid out a list of everything you should have.

Chapter 1 – Pack's

As the title of this book suggests, it's all about the kit and what you put inside it. If your kit is large enough, you can call it a pack. While you can spend a fair amount of money on advanced kits, a better strategy would be to either start from scratch or with a bare bone first aid kit and then supplement the kit with additional supplies.

For starters, you should have more than one kit. I recommend at least three, one for your home, one for your car or bike, and then one to take on your person in case you go hiking or will be an extended distance from your home or transportation. If you want just one kit, you should then pick a large pack for the home, which should have a smaller portable pack for your car, and yet an even smaller kit which you can remove to take on foot. Regardless of how you organize them, each of the smaller kits should still contain most of the same components just fewer of each item.

The thing about prepackaged kits or packs is that they are typically designed for specific circumstances. Some are more geared towards tending wounds, others are more focused on food and surviving the wild. To be fully prepared you'll need a bit of everything. As such, one strategy would be to buy three different basic kits for three different scenarios, and then borrow from each. You can then supplement each of the three with additional supplies. If you are starting from scratch, you will simply add more supplies of each item in your larger kits.

For packs stored on your person and in your car or bike, you want to make sure they are made of light and durable materials. Waterproof and sun proof material is also highly recommended. Larger packs stored in your home can be heavier and don't necessarily need to be sun proof, but they should be waterproof in the event of a flood.

Your packs should also include a checklist, preferably on the outside, but if not, you should have a checklist easily accessible on a secured pocket or lining on the inside, and your supplies should be dated. Dating your supplies is essential so you can prevent expired medicine or food. Even tools should be dated and periodically replaced from time to time.

Once your packs are fully stocked with supplies, which we'll discuss more in detail in further chapters, you should check your pack at a minimum of four times per year or once per quarter. This is to make sure you have all the supplies you need and that your supplies are still good and useful, but regardless of where you are with money or supplies, the main thing is to get started even if that means starting with just a waterproof zip lock bag with a few essentials.

Chapter 2 – Tools

For starters, I highly recommend a Swiss army knife. A basic pocket knife may work for your personal kit, but the one in your car or bike should have a multi-functional knife for multiple purposes. This is like having your own utility belt in a much smaller space. It will be invaluable for many unforeseen circumstances. A manual food can opener should also be included if your Swiss army or pocket knife doesn't contain that feature.

Make sure that your knife is legal in your jurisdiction. When using the actual blade, always cut away from yourself and others. Knives can be used not only as a weapon but also for things such as cutting ropes and bandages, opening things, making a fire (bow drill), cutting branches and tarp for shelters, and numerous other things.

You should also have a compass or other tool for navigation. Smart phones with GPS apps will do you no good if cell towers are down. A basic compass and a physical map of your area plus a national map are needed.

You should also include a method to contact someone in case of an emergency. Again, if you cell phone is not working for whatever reason, signal flares will be essential. For smaller kits, a reflecting mirror and a whistle can work as well. I recommend all three. Also add glow sticks for visibility in the dark.

Your pack at home or in your car should include WD-40. Your personal pack should include some type of non-oil based lubricant. This is extremely helpful if you find yourself stuck or you have a mechanical device that is stuck and immobile.

In addition, you should have fish hooks and a sewing kit. You will have numerous uses for these besides fishing or sewing. They can be used for medical purposes as well as retrieving items.

A solar powered battery recharger is important for your two larger kits. You should also have solar powered or hand powered flashlights and radios. A disposable cell phone or solar powered recharger with an adapter for your cell phone is also recommended. There are various methods of making your own if you are unable to find one that is ready made. Just be sure that you check to make sure that it works before you add it to your kit.

Duct tape is another must. This tool has a seemingly infinite number of uses. Don't leave home without it. Just make sure that your tape, like everything else, has been dated. It won't do you any good if it's no longer sticky.

Hollow tubing is also helpful. I would include different sizes, both narrow and wide. Narrow tubing can be used to open up airways in cases of blockages from food. It can also be used to create makeshift intravenous bags to deliver food, water and medicine.

Wider tubing can be used to transport gas, oil, water, and other liquids. It can be used as a makeshift underwater breathing apparatus or to ventilate an area or siphon air through a small space.

A rescue tool is also useful, especially in cars. These can be used to cut seat belts and break glass in the event of an accident or submersion under water. In cars, a jack and spare tire are also necessary. Those along with jumper cables should be in every car.

I would also include a basic tool kit. You can find small multifunctional kits that contain things like hammers and screwdrivers. You should also make sure you have nails and screws as well. A nail gun and stapler are also handy, both of which have medical and protective applications. Include a plunger, and insect bait. You'll be surprised at the applications of both.

Finally, you should have a survival manual. It may sound silly, but it could save your life. Have one for your home and car, and a mini packet for your personal kit. It's a great idea to actually read the guides prior to adding them, but no one has a perfect memory, so find a good guide and bring it with you. If you're out of cell range and you need it, you'll thank yourself that you did when the time comes.

Chapter 3 – Medicine

You can't have a survival medical kit without medicine and first aid, so here we go. I will only briefly reference items mentioned in other section for medical uses, starting with duct tape.

Duct tape can be used to close a wound, among other things. To go with the duct tape, you should have something that you can use to suture the wound first, namely, butterfly sutures. If you have a large cut or gash, this is a great way to close the wound temporarily until you can reach a hospital to see if you need real stitches. For smaller cuts, this may be all you need to close the wound. Just make sure that you clean the wound first with water and alcohol or disinfectants.

You should also have absorbent compress dressings, at least two for each kit. Too much moisture can lead to infection, so after the wounded is cleaned and disinfected, make sure you absorb any excess moisture, which can also weaken adhesive seals from bandages.

Make sure you have plenty of bandages. At least 25 in various sizes and shapes are recommended by the Red Cross. I would include at least twice that many so you have separate them for your portable kits. You should also include two three inches and two four-inch roller bandages for larger wounds.

That brings us to a very important section, which is disinfectants and infection preventions. Soap and water is the minimum you need to clean a wound, and this should be included in your kit, but you should also have either alcohol or peroxide. Antiseptic wipes are an excellent option, especially for smaller kits. Still, I would include alcohol in at least your home kit. I also recommend antiseptic creams, which you can apply periodically and can speed up healing.

You should also have something to cover the wound such as gauze. Smaller band aids are also useful, but medical gauze is more effective for the larger wounds. You should also include quick clotting gauze. This will aid in clotting for cuts and gashes. Other sections also mentioned coverings, such as bandanas, which can be used in a pinch if you are out of gauze or missing it for some reason. Other coverings may work as well if you have no other option.

Other guides may recommend trying to get an advance prescription of antibiotics, but I recommend against this. This is the sort of thing that has created antibiotic resistant strains of bacteria, and you also do not have the medical expertise to decide if you need one or which type would be preferred. Stick with prevention on this count.

I would also recommend against any other prescription medication, with the exception of making sure you have an existing supply of any long term prescription drugs you may be taking. Stick with the over the counter medication. Keep it safe, and keep it legal.

Also, don't fall into the trap of natural or homeopathic medicine. That isn't real medication, and it won't help you one bit if you need something in an emergency. Natural medications are also not uniform in their ingredients, the amount of the ingredients, and can have interactions with other drugs. Stick with what is supported by evidence based science. That doesn't mean you can used herbs in the wild. If you are aware of specific drugs or substances contained in plants that are scientifically supported to improve or aid in healing, such as aloe vera, feel free to use them in you have access.

What you should have is lot of over the counter medication, which I'll discuss in a moment. You should also be aware of any allergies as well as common side effects or interactions between various drugs as well as any prescription drugs you may be taking. It may be a good idea to look up the medications ahead of time so you can select types that you know will not interact with any drugs you are taking now.

Along those lines, I would also include a medical manual for emergencies. Your survival manual, which you should have as well, will cover some basics, but I would add a specific one for medicine. Again, you may not feel the need to take a paper manual in lieu of a digital version, but you may not also have access to a fully charged phone or electronic device, so don't skimp on this one.

The first type of medication you should have is pain medication. As mentioned before, stick with the legal variety. Aleve, Aspirin, Tylenol, and Ibuprofen are a must. Aleve works great, but if something works better for you, feel free to include that as well.

For muscle pain, cold and heat pads work great. They've already been mentioned in other sections, so you should have them on hand. You can also include muscle cream for additional relief if that works better for you. I would also add skin creams, such as hydrocortisone as well as topical anesthetics, such as oral gel, for dental or oral relief. You should also include Calamine lotion for rashes. Don't forget to throw in insect repellant as well.

Another category of drugs you should include is antihistamines for allergies. You can add something like Benadryl, but I would also include something for severe allergic reactions such as an EpiPen for things like nut, shellfish, or bee allergies.

Burns are another category that you should be prepared for. I would include both sunscreen, but prevention of sunburns, as well as aloe vera gels for sun damage and general skin healing. You should also have medicated burn creams for more severe first and second degree burns.

In addition, make sure you include stomach and digestive medications such as anti-diarrhea medication, laxatives, antacids, anti-nausea, and anti-gas meds. Pepto-Bismol is a good all-around stomach medication, but include whatever you prefer.

Anti-cold medications should also be included. Add items such as decongestants as well as fever and cough suppressants. Nighttime and daytime options are a plus.

You should also be prepared for fractures and broken bones. In the tools and ropes section, you should have netting or ropes that can be used for setting and tying, but you should also include some inexpensive SAM splints which are often used by emergency medical personnel.

You should have a Swiss Army knife, or at least a pocket knife. Check to see if you have tweezers or nail clippers included in the knife. If not, stock them separately.

A few additional items include a stethoscope, scalpel, needles and syringe, ear or bulb syringe (for cleaning out the nose or earwax), thermometer, Q-tips, eyewash and dressing, safety pins, cotton balls, as well as grooming supplies.

One important thing to remember about the medical section of your kit is that your items should be dated. You may not need to write the date on the items themselves, but you should have an insert with each category dated so you can periodically replace expired and old items. Medicine does expire. It can lose its effectiveness and even break down chemically into other substances, with can create other side effects or interactions.

Also, make sure you have three sets of medical supplies, one for your larger home kit, as well as one for your car or bike and one for your person. That means at a minimum, you should have three of each item or three items for the same purpose, which you can separate into smaller sections as needed.

I would also recommend that you education yourself in first aid. Learn how to do basic CPR and the Heimlich maneuver. Read and review your first aid kit and medical manual so you are familiar with it and know where to find it quickly if you need to brush up on the specifics.

Finally, make sure you have copies of any relevant medical consent forms and something to write with. Hopefully you won't need to use this, but include them anyway just in case.

Chapter 4 – Ropes

Ropes can be used for a variety of things. They can be used in conjunction with a bandana as a tourniquet. They allow you to climb or descend obstacles for movement or escape. Ropes can hold you in place during a flood, prevent you from falling, or rescue others. They can hoist objects, be used for hunting, kindling, signaling, or numerous other purposes including medical applications such as setting a fracture.

Survival rope packs can be purchased for as little as five dollars. Be careful though, because different ropes do different things, so you need to educate yourself one which type of rope is best for certain situations such as strength, water resistance, weight, etc. I recommend more than one type of rope. A combination of two or three ropes is preferable.

Of all the ropes, you should include paracord (used in parachutes) as your primary rope. Include this no matter what. It is extremely lightweight, durable, strong, an versatile, which is the key in any survival event.

Paracord can serve the function of hiking, building traps, fishing, holding or securing gear, tying a tarp, sewing, trip wire, flossing, creating a pulley, sling, catapult, building a ladder or hammock, making a raft, be used as a bow drill for a fire, repairing broken equipment, making shelter, or making a stretcher.

Like many things, though, you get what you pay for. Make sure you invest in quality paracord. When the time comes, you'll be grateful that you did.

Good secondary ropes can include things like bungee cord, climbing ropes, or tow straps (not actually a rope, but should be included in your car nonetheless).

Make sure that at a minimum, you include paracord in your car and home kits, and include more than one type of rope if you can.

Chapter 5 – Coverage

There are several items that should be included for coverage. The first is trash bags. These can be used as ponchos, storage, or other purposes. If you have a bright colored bag, such as the orange versions used by the transportation department, that's even better.

Another coverage item that should be included is a light-weight foil space blanket. This will be used for warmth as well as sleeping or hiding.

A bandana is also a surprisingly useful survival tool. They can do more than just hold your hair in place. They can keep you warm, work as a placeholder, carry items, be used as tinder or kindling for a fire, soak up water or sweat, alert others to an emergency, filter water, make a waste bag, be used as a bandage, extend cords, clean, block the sun, be used as a mask, mark trails, hold pots, or even be used as a weapon.

I would also include a hat. While you can use a bandana to cover your head, a separate hat should be included as coverage from the sun, wind, and rain. You may need the bandana for something else. Sunglasses and face paint should also be include for camouflage and protection against the elements.

You should also add an extra change of clothes. This should be self-explanatory. Add a pair of gloves as well. Surgical gloves should be in your personal pack, but your larger packs should include larger gloves for warmth or manual tasks.

In addition, I would include a water proof mat, such as a yoga matt. This can be used as insulation or to block smoke. A fabric blanket or towel should also be included, which can be used for warmth, to soak up water, as a partition, or an additional filter. It can also be used as additional kindling.

Another set of items you should include are absorbent pads for children, female needs, and the elderly. Be well stocked on these in cased of a prolonged period without access to a store or residence.

Shelter is another consideration, especially if you are injured or in extreme cold, heat, wind, dust, or other harsh weather. You can make your own make shift shelter with the items already discussed here and in earlier sections. Your trash bags and paracord could be used as a basic tarp or tent. Just make sure that you do a bit of research beforehand so you know how you can efficiently set it up.

Chapter 6 – Fire

Start with a magnifying glass. You can heat up paper and dry materials by concentrating the suns energy without the need for matches. This will be invaluable if you run out of matches or your matches get wet.

Matches are still useful, so add them too. I also recommend a big shot butane torch for your larger packs. This will come in handy for protection and hunting when you run out of food. This also means stocking up on a bit of butane. Start with a lighter for your smaller packs, but then work up to the butane torch for your car and home packs.

In addition, you should have some tinder or materials that can be used to set fire. Don't assume you'll always have materials from your environment. Without something that can be burned, there is no fire. If your emergency kit in your home or car is well stocked, you should also have additional items which can be used as kindling, such as a fabric blanket or towel, bandana, or spare clothes.

Smoke from fire can also be used for different things such as signaling for help. In addition, smoke can paralyze certain insects and wild creatures, such as certain bees or wasps.

You should also be prepared to not just start a fire, but escape from one. This means, you can use those same fabrics used for kindling as face masks. They can also be used to absorb water and keep you and your area damp if needed.

Protective goggles or glasses can also be used to protect your used in the event you need to make or escape from a fire. A fire blanket and mini fire-extinguisher should also be included in your auto or home kit.

Chapter 7 – Food & Water

Water and food are essential to survival, and you should have them in all your kits, including your personal kit. You should also have a plan to get more food and purify water if your existing supplies run out.

Water is more important than food, but clean water is even more important. This means you need purification tablets. You can treat at much as 25 quarts with a single bottle of the iodine based variety.

Another option would be a small amount of unscented bleach. A couple drops can purify a liter of water. There is a problem with bleach, though, in that it degrades over time. A better chemical is calcium hypochlorite. A one-pound bag of the stuff can purify 10,000 gallons of water and is more effective at killing other types of pathogens. The process is more involved, and I would only recommend it for your larger household kit. UV lighting devices, such as UVSteripen, can also disinfect water and cost as little as $40.

A portable filter is also useful if you can't use the above methods. You can find simple techniques to use coffee filters, crushed charcoal, small sand or pebbles, and then larger gravel in a water bottle or other container to quickly filter water in a rush.

The fall back, however, is always boiling water. If you have a way to heat up water with fire, such as matches or a magnifying glass, boil your water to kill bacteria, parasites, and other pathogens. Boiling water is the single most effective way to purify water. It won't, however, get rid of salt or heavy metals unless you use condensation capture methods after boiling. If you think your water may have lead, mercury, or other contaminants, I recommend using a filter prior to boiling, or desalinate your water by capturing condensation if you are getting water from the sea.

An emergency supply of food should be included in every kit. Start with the basics, freeze dried food packets with something that can make fire. Fire was already discussed in an earlier section of the book, but it will be very important if you find yourself in a situation where you are forced to find food beyond your existing supplies. Thoroughly cooking wild game will insure that you won't contract most diseases and infections.

Still, there are other options for food. A few protein or energy bars is a good start for a mini pack on the go, at least in the beginning. You can also find a 30 day supply of vitamin and mineral supplements for the food storage for as little as $30. This won't contain and the protein and sugars you'll need, but will give you the minimum necessary to keep going once your supply stock has run out. Hopefully by that time, you will have been rescued. If not, it will give you plenty of time and find or hunt for more food in the interim.

You should also add cold and heat packets. You can find light, cheap chemical packets which can be used not only for heating or cooling food and water, but they can also be used as cold and hot compresses for medical purposes.

A final discussion on food should also include what to do in the event that you find yourself with no supplies. In that instance, you want will need to find or hunt for food. The first rule of eating in the wild is not to eat something unless you are absolutely sure you know what it is. If you know the area, and are certain what you are eating is blackberries as opposed to poison berries of some variety you'll have an advantage. If you are unsure, follow the recommendations in the next paragraph.

If you are near a body of water, fishing can also be a life saver. Netting and capture methods may be more effective in the long term, but if you've stock the fish hook and thread, as recommended in earlier chapters, you'll have what you need to catch fish.

Skimming, filtering, and drying kelp or seaweed is an excellent way to supplement your food supply. They are high in many nutrients and will go a long way in providing you a long term food source if you need it.

If you must survive away from a body of water, eating higher on the food chain may save your life, but stick to small game. Small game requires less energy and is far safer than running around like a maniac trying to trap or spear wild bears deer.

If there are no plants that you know are edible, insects are never in short supply. Insects will supply you with the protein you need to keep going, and if you're well stocked on a 30-day supplement of vitamins and minerals you'll be in decent shape. Also, if you've stocked the recommended items in prior sections, you'll have all that you need to acquire insects and small game such as rabbits, raccoons, or squirrels. Usually, though, all you need to capture insects is a stick or a little bit of elbow grease.

Unless you are an expert on fruits and berries, I would skip the berries and go straight to finding nuts. Tree nuts provide an excellent source of fats and protein. To list a few, there are acorns, beechnuts, chestnuts, black walnuts, butternuts, and hickory nuts to name a few. The flavor can vary from tree to tree, and I recommend roasting them. Still, tree nuts can harbor hidden dangers. There are a few toxic nuts, such as the nut from the buckeye tree. One might also have allergic reactions to certain nuts, so make sure you know your allergies, and inform yourself on the nuts in your area.

Finally, I would include some type of container. Something like a hydro flask would work great, but you might want to include a bowl, utensils, and power towels as well.

Conclusion

Regardless of the situation, planning is always essential. The most basic planning is what you need to do before you are in a situation where you or a loved one are in an emergency. Whether it's preparation for a natural disaster, or something else, plan ahead by taking a few short steps to stock a basic medicine kit. That, along with the knowledge of first aid might save your life in many situations.

Make sure that your emergency kit includes smaller portable sub kits that can be used in your car and on your person. Educate yourself on how to use the items you have, and check often to make sure that your perishables are still good. While this may not save you in every instance, it will maximize your chances to survive as much as possible, which is all you can hope for.

As with most situations, a little preparation goes a long way. More importantly, the best advice I can give is to remain calm and conserve energy wherever possible. This will help prevent you from doing silly things and making stupid mistakes in the event of an emergency. It will also extend the time you need to survive or get rescued. Having a well-stocked emergency kit can only assist in that endeavor, so long as you know where it is at all times and that your kit is out of the reach of children.

FREE Bonus Reminder

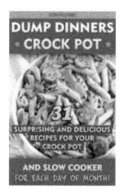

If you have not grabbed it yet, please go ahead and download your Free Ebook *"Dump Dinners Crock Pot: 31 Surprising And Delicious Recipes For Your Crock Pot And Slow Cooker For Each Day of Month!"*

Simply Click the Button Below

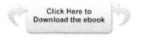

OR **Go to This Page**

http://easycookingideas.com/free

BONUS #2: More Free & Discounted Books

Do you want to receive more Free & Discounted Books?

We have a mailing list where we send out our new Books when they go free or with a discount on Kindle. Click on the link below to sign up for Free & Discount Book Promotions.

=> Sign Up for Free & Discount Book Promotions <=

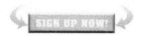

OR Go to this URL

http://zbit.ly/1WBb1Ek

www.ingramcontent.com/pod-product-compliance
Lightning Source LLC
LaVergne TN
LVHW011048220225
804319LV00010B/879